MANAGING PRINGLES DISEASE

Uncovering the Mystery of Pringles Disease: Understanding Its Cause and Potential Treatments

By

Kelvin Jason

Table of Contents

Copyright © by Dr. Kelvin Jason 2024. All rights reserved.

Chapter 1

Introduction to Pringle's disease

Pringle's disease is a rare condition that affects the liver. It is characterized by a narrowing of the hepatic artery, which is the main artery that supplies blood to the liver. This narrowing can cause a decrease in blood flow to the liver, which can lead to liver damage.

Pringles Disease is an often under-recognized, but serious, respiratory illness caused by exposure to asbestos dust in the workplace. It was first reported in the United Kingdom in the late 1970s, when an employee at a manufacturing plant in Carlisle was diagnosed with the disease after being exposed to asbestos fibers during the manufacturing process.

Pringles Disease is caused by inhalation of dust particles containing asbestos fibers, which can irritate the lungs and cause inflammation. The asbestos fibers damage the lungs over time, leading to a progressive loss of lung function. Symptoms can include coughing, shortness of breath, and chest pain. In more severe cases, pleurisy and fluid accumulation in the lungs may also occur.

What is Pringle's disease?

Pringle's disease is named after Sir John Pringle, a Scottish surgeon who first described the condition in 1750. Pringle's disease is also known as hepatic artery stenosis or hepatic artery narrowing.

Symptoms of Pringle's disease

The symptoms of Pringle's disease can vary depending on the severity of the narrowing of the hepatic artery. Some people with Pringle's disease may have no symptoms at all.

Others may experience symptoms such as:

1. Pain in the upper right abdomen

2. Nausea and vomiting

3. Fatigue

4. Jaundice

5. Fever

6. Weight loss

Causes of Pringle's Disease

The cause of Pringle's disease is unknown in most cases. However, it is possibly caused by a combination of genetic and environmental factors.

Some of the factors that may increase the risk of developing Pringle's disease include:

1. Age
2. Gender (men are more likely to develop Pringle's disease than women)
3. Family history of Pringle's disease
4. Certain medical conditions, such as atherosclerosis (hardening of the arteries) and inflammatory bowel disease
5. Smoking
6. Alcohol use

Pringle's disease is a rare childhood disorder that is caused by mutations in the gene that codes for fibroblast growth factor 20 (FGF20). This gene is responsible for controlling the growth and development of cells in the central nervous system. The most common cause of the disorder is a mutation that results in an abnormal form of FGF20 production.

MANAGING PRINGLES DISEASE

In some cases, Pringle's disease can be caused by a spontaneous mutation in a gene other than FGF20. Mutations in other genes, such as those involved in neuron development and metabolism, can also cause the disorder. Additionally, environmental factors, such as exposure to toxic substances, may also contribute to Pringle's disease.

Pringle's disease typically manifests as a combination of neurological and muscular symptoms. The neurological symptoms include poor muscle coordination, spasticity, and delayed development. The muscular symptoms range from mild to severe forms of muscular atrophy, which can cause muscle weakness and loss of coordination.

The precise cause of Pringle's disease is not yet known. The genetic and environmental components of the disorder are both being studied in order to provide insight into its cause. Research is ongoing and new treatments are being developed in an effort to improve the lives of those affected by Pringle's disease.

Today, Pringle's disease is a relatively rare condition, but it is still extremely important to be aware of its signs and symptoms in order to provide the best possible care for those affected.

The exact cause of Pringle's disease is still not fully understood. However, according to current research, the condition is associated with FGF20 mutations and the disruption of cell growth and development in the central nervous system. Additional research is ongoing to help determine its other causes and possible treatments.

It is important to note that Pringle's disease can vary greatly in its severity and symptoms. Therefore, it is highly recommended that those affected seek medical assistance in order to receive the best possible care.

By understanding the causes of Pringle's disease, medical professionals will be able to develop better ways to diagnose and treat the condition. This will improve the quality of life for those affected by Pringle's disease and will help to ensure that more effective treatments are available in the future.

Story

Monica had just been diagnosed with Pringles Disease, a rare and untreatable neurological disorder. She was understandably devastated. She had read all the medical literature on the disease and knew that there was no known cure, only palliative treatments that could give her relief for a period of time.

MANAGING PRINGLES DISEASE

Monica was determined to find a way to recover from Pringles Disease. She researched every possible treatment and talked to numerous doctors, trying to find a solution. Finally, she found a doctor who said he had seen some success with a specific combination of medications.

Monica began taking the prescribed medications and started to notice a difference within a few weeks. Gradually, her symptoms began to improve and she regained her mobility and started to regain her energy. She eventually made a full recovery and was able to live her life without any major lifestyle changes.

Monica was so thankful to the doctor and the medications that she credits for her recovery. Now she is an advocate for the disease and talks to anyone she can about the importance of early diagnosis and treatment. She is hopeful that her story will be an inspiration to others and help to spread awareness about the disease.Monica's story shows that with the right medications, Pringles Disease can be reversed. She is a living testament that no matter how bleak the situation seems, there is always hope.

Chapter 2

Preventing Pringles Disease

There is no sure way to prevent Pringle's disease. However, there are some things you can do to reduce your risk of developing the condition. These include:

1. Eat a healthy diet.

2. Exercise regularly.

3. Don't smoke.

4. Limit alcohol use.

5. Control your blood pressure and cholesterol levels.

Healthy Diet for Pringles Disease

A healthy diet for Pringles disease is one that prioritizes getting plenty of vitamins, minerals, and essential fatty acids from plant-based sources. It should also focus on avoiding high-calorie, processed, and unhealthy foods that may have a negative impact on Pringle's disease symptoms.

For optimal health, individuals with Pringle's disease should strive to eat a diverse mix of nutrient-rich whole foods like fruits, vegetables, whole grains, beans, nuts, and seeds. These foods should have plenty of vitamins, minerals, fiber, and Omega-3 fatty acids, which are essential for healthy immune function. It is also important to choose organic when possible to avoid artificial chemicals and pesticides.

When it comes to proteins, lean meats, such as fish, chicken, and turkey, are good options. Other animal proteins, such as dairy and eggs, should be consumed in moderation as they can provide too much-saturated fat. Plant-based proteins, such as legumes, nuts, and seeds, are excellent sources of healthy proteins and should be included.

It is also important to focus on limiting unhealthy fats found in processed foods and deep-fried items. Instead, opt for healthier fats such as monounsaturated fats (found in avocados, nuts, and olives) and polyunsaturated fats (found in fatty fish, vegetable oils, and nuts).

Overall, the aim should be to consume a balanced diet that is rich in vitamins, minerals, and essential fatty acids. By eating a variety of nutrient-dense, plant-based foods and limiting unhealthy fats, individuals with Pringles disease can improve their condition and overall health.

Regular Exercise for Pringles disease

Regular exercise has been shown to be beneficial for people suffering from Pringles Disease. Pringles Disease, also known as Pseudo-Keratolysis Solare, is a skin condition that results in the development of a dry, scaly skin patch on the outer surface of the cheeks, usually following sun exposure. Regular exercise can reduce the symptoms associated with Pringles Disease.

Regular exercise can help improve blood flow to the affected area, which will help reduce the symptoms. Improved blood flow assists in better skin cell regeneration and healing and can help reduce the scaling, itching, and redness associated with Pringles Disease. Additionally, exercise can help diminish inflammation, which can reduce redness, pain, and discomfort.

Regular exercise also boosts the production of endorphins, natural hormones that make you feel good. Endorphins help reduce stress and elevate mood, which can be beneficial for someone dealing with this skin condition. Additionally, regular exercise can help build strength, increase flexibility, and improve balance and coordination, enabling Pringles sufferers to remain mobile and active.

Exercising at home is a great way to get regular activity when dealing with Pringles Disease. Low-impact exercises, such as stretching and yoga, are beneficial as they are gentle on the skin and can be done without too much physical strain. Walking, jogging, and swimming are also great exercises that can help promote circulation and reduce inflammation.

Incorporating regular exercise into your routine is beneficial for anyone suffering from Pringles Disease. Regular physical activity can help reduce symptoms, improve blood flow, and boost overall mood, allowing individuals to remain active and stay healthy.

Avoid Excessive Alcohol Consumption for Pringles Disease.

Pringles Disease is the informal name for a condition caused by excessive alcohol consumption. Pringles Disease is also referred to as "alcoholic myopathy," a type of muscle weakness that often affects the arms and legs. It is believed to be brought on by the damaging effects of alcohol on muscle tissues.

Alcohol is a toxic substance that can damage your body if consumed in excessive amounts. Excessive alcohol consumption can lead to a number of serious health issues including Pringles Disease. As such, it is important to limit your consumption of alcohol in order to remain healthy.

You should first limit your consumption of alcoholic beverages each day and consider avoiding it altogether if possible. If you have to drink, then ensure that you do so in moderation. This includes avoiding binge drinking or consuming drinks in excess of the recommended safe limit. In addition to this, be sure to drink a glass of water in between each alcoholic drink this can help to reduce your alcohol consumption. Also, try to have a healthy diet that consists of fresh fruits and vegetables as well as lean proteins. A balanced diet not only helps to combat intoxication but also helps to reduce your risk of developing Pringles Disease.

Exercising regularly is also an effective way of reducing your alcohol consumption. Regular physical activity can help to reduce the cravings associated with drinking and can also maintain your overall health. It is also important to remain hydrated by drinking plenty of water throughout the day in order to prevent dehydration, a common side effect of heavy drinking.

It is possible to reduce the chances of developing Pringles Disease by limiting your alcohol consumption. You should remain aware of how much you are drinking and ensure that you are not consuming more than the recommended safe limits. By following these tips and taking regular preventive care of your body, you can live a healthy lifestyle and reduce your risk of alcohol-related issues, such as Pringles Disease.

Avoid smoking for Pringles disease

Pringles disease, also known as distal radius fracture, is a common bone break at the end of the arm near the wrist. It can be painful and disabling, and in some cases, may require surgery. One way to reduce your risk of Pringles disease is to avoid smoking.

Smoking has been linked to a variety of health risks, including Pringles disease. Studies have shown that the risk of Pringles disease is significantly higher in people who smoke, compared to those who don't. Smoking decreases blood circulation to the bones, depriving them of nutrients and oxygen that they need to remain healthy. This can lead to weakened bones, making them more susceptible to breaks.

In addition to increasing the risk of Pringles disease, smoking also decreases the effectiveness of any treatment that may be used to correct the fracture. This means that smoking not only increases the risk of getting Pringles disease, but can also make it harder to fully recover.

If you are currently a smoker, quitting smoking is the best way to reduce your risk of Pringles disease. In addition to quitting, reducing your risk for Pringles disease may include practicing safety techniques while participating in sports, wearing protective gear when possible, and addressing any nutritional deficiencies.

Pringles disease is a serious condition that can cause pain and disability. To reduce the chances of getting Pringles disease, avoid smoking and practice safety techniques. Doing so can help keep your bones strong and healthy, and decrease your risk of developing Pringles disease.

Controlling blood pressure and cholesterol levels for Pringles disease

Pringles disease, also known as hyperlipidemia, is a medical condition characterized by abnormally high levels of certain lipids (fats) in the blood. High levels of these lipids can lead to an increased risk of cardiovascular disease, stroke, and even heart attack. People with Pringles disease are at higher risk of developing cardiovascular disease, so it is important for them to take steps to control their blood pressure and cholesterol levels. Monitoring and controlling blood pressure and cholesterol levels is critical for people living with Pringles disease. Blood pressure should be checked at least twice a year, and cholesterol levels should be monitored at least once a year. It is important to take steps to reduce your risk of cardiovascular disease by making lifestyle changes.

Healthy eating, getting regular physical activity, limiting alcohol consumption, quitting smoking, and reducing stress can help to reduce blood pressure and cholesterol levels. Maintaining a healthy diet is key in controlling blood pressure and cholesterol levels. Eating plenty of fruits, vegetables, and whole grains, while limiting unhealthy fats and simple sugars can help to reduce cholesterol levels. It is also important to get enough omega-3 fatty acids, which have been proven to reduce inflammation and lower cholesterol levels. Additionally, avoiding foods like meats with high levels of saturated fat can help lower cholesterol levels and reduce the risk of cardiovascular disease.

Taking necessary medications is also critical for controlling blood pressure and cholesterol levels in people with Pringles disease. Medications, such as statins, can be prescribed to lower cholesterol levels. Blood pressure medications can also be prescribed to reduce hypertension and keep blood pressure levels in the healthy range.

Controlling blood pressure and cholesterol levels is an essential part of managing Pringles disease. Making lifestyle changes, monitoring blood pressure and cholesterol levels, and taking medications as prescribed can help reduce the risk of cardiovascular disease in people with this condition. **If you have any concerns about your risk of developing Pringle's disease, talk to your doctor.**

They can help you assess your risk and make recommendations for reducing it.

Chapter 3

Diagnosing Pringle's Disease

Pringle's Disease, also known as pleuropulmonary lithiasis, is a rare lung disorder in which calcium and other minerals form deposits in the lungs. It is often asymptomatic and a diagnosis is usually made when an abnormality in the lungs is seen on an imaging test.

The main diagnostic tool used to diagnose Pringle's Disease is chest radiography. This imaging test uses X-rays to create images of the chest and lungs that can be examined for abnormalities. If abnormalities are found, a computed tomography (CT) scan or magnetic resonance imaging (MRI) can then be done to confirm the diagnosis.

Since Pringle's Disease is asymptomatic, it can be easily missed upon diagnosis, especially if imaging tests are not taken. It is important for physicians to be aware of this disorder and to consider it when considering the diagnosis of a lung disorder. If symptoms of Pringle's Disease are present, a bronchoscopy may be performed where a scope is inserted into the airway to examine the trachea and bronchi for deposits.

Pringle's Disease is a rare disorder, but its diagnosis is important in order to provide proper treatment to prevent further complications. Diagnosis of Pringle's Disease requires a comprehensive approach that should include a thorough physical examination, a review of symptoms, and confirming imaging tests for accurate diagnosis. Through this approach, Pringle's Disease can be identified and managed appropriately, allowing for improved quality of life and improved health outcomes overall.

Chapter 4

Treatments for Pringle's Disease

Pringle's Disease, also known as sclerosing cholangitis, is a rare form of chronic inflammation of the bile ducts. It is a progressive and potentially life-threatening condition that can lead to severe bile duct damage, liver failure, and other complications.

Treatment for Pringle's Disease usually involves lifestyle changes, medications, and/or surgery.

Medications for Pringles patients

The most commonly prescribed medications for Pringle's patient (a patient suffering from a condition called Pringle's Syndrome, characterized by chronic pain and depression) are generally antidepressants and mood stabilizers. These can include medications like selective serotonin reuptake inhibitors (SSRIs) such as Lexapro, Zoloft, and Prozac, and serotonin-norepinephrine reuptake inhibitors (SNRIs) such as Cymbalta. Mood stabilizers like Depakote, Lamictal and Lithium may also be prescribed.

In addition to these medications, patients may also benefit from other medications to treat specific symptoms.

For example, for those with sleep disturbances, medications like trazodone, temazepam, and zolpidem can help improve sleep. For those with severe depression and/or symptoms of anxiety, anti-anxiety medications like benzodiazepines (Xanax, Ativan, etc.) may also be prescribed.

In order to ensure that medications are as effective as possible, it is important that Pringle's patients are also provided with psychological treatments to help them manage their condition. Psychotherapy and cognitive behavioral therapy can help patients gain an understanding of their condition and how to better cope with symptoms. This, in turn, can help reduce the potential side effects of medications and make them more effective.

Finally, it is important for patients with Pringle's Syndrome to maintain a healthy lifestyle. This includes making sure to eat a balanced diet, exercising regularly, and getting enough rest and sleep. Patients should also ensure that they get emotional support from friends and family as this can help them better cope with and manage their condition.

Surgery for pringles patient

Surgery might be an option for an individual diagnosed with pringles disease, depending on their specific needs and the severity of their symptoms. Surgery is considered when other treatments, such as physical therapy and medications, have been unsuccessful in alleviating pringles symptoms. If surgery is recommended, the type and extent of the procedure is determined on a case-by-case basis.

Some invasive surgeries that may be considered include carpal tunnel release, extensor retinaculum release, cubital tunn el release, and ganglionectomy. During a carpal tunnel release, the surgeon may make a small incision in the wrist to gain access to the underside of the transverse carpal ligament. This ligament is released to relieve pressure on the median nerve and reduce the pain and discomfort associated with the condition. Similarly, an extensor retinaculum release involves creating an incision in the wrist to access the extensor retinacular sheath, which is then cut or removed to reduce pressure on the median nerve. Other potentially recommended surgeries include cubital tunnel release, which involves gaining access to the ulnar nerve and releasing it, as well as ganglionectomy, which is the surgical removal of a ganglion cyst that is causing nerve compression.

In some cases, minimally invasive, endoscopic surgery may be recommended. This type of surgery is performed using a thin tube with a camera and tools at the end. The camera is used to gain a better view of the affected area, and the tools are used to cut or remove part of the tissue or muscle that's exerting pressure on the nerves.

No matter what type of procedure is recommended, the primary goal is to reduce the pressure on the nerves and associated painful symptoms. If surgery is deemed necessary, the patient's physician may order pre-operative testing and provide post-operative instructions before the surgery is scheduled. After the procedure is completed, the patient may require physical therapy and follow-up care to achieve full recovery.

Making lifestyle changes, such as limiting what you eat and avoiding alcohol, can help prevent or reduce flares and reduce symptoms. Medications, such as antibiotics, corticosteroids, and immunosuppressants, can also help reduce inflammation and improve symptoms. Surgery, such as stenting or a liver transplant, can be used to correct bile duct damage and improve symptoms.

In addition to lifestyle changes, medications, and surgery, some alternative therapies have been shown to be beneficial for people with Pringle's Disease. Some of these therapies include stress management, acupuncture, yoga, massage, herbal supplements, and Chinese herbal remedies.

It is important to talk to your doctor before trying any type of alternative therapy. Be sure to consult your doctor for complete information about treatment options for Pringle's Disease.

Chapter 5

Long-Term Outlook for Pringle's Disease

The long-term outlook for patients with Pringle's Disease is generally favorable. With proper medical care, patients can experience an improvement in their symptoms and quality of life. Pringle's Disease is a chronic condition, which means that symptoms may come and go over time, but with proper care and treatment, many patients are able to enjoy a normal life.

In some cases, surgery may be useful in easing symptoms and reducing the risk of complications. Surgery may be an option for people who haven't responded to other treatments or whose Pringle's Disease is causing serious problems. Surgery can help to reduce the size of the artery wall, reduce the risk of rupture, and decrease the risk of stroke.

People with Pringle's Disease also need to manage their risk factors for heart disease, such as smoking, high blood pressure, and diabetes. Regular exercise, a healthy diet, and stress management are all important components of managing Pringle's Disease. It is also important to monitor for other conditions, such as high cholesterol or heart rhythm disturbances, that may contribute to Pringle's Disease.

The outlook for people with Pringle's Disease continues to improve as new treatments are developed and old treatments are refined. With careful management, many patients can experience a good quality of life and relatively few complications if they remain vigilant about their lifestyle choices.

Chapter 6

Resources for Pringles Disease

Pringles Disease, more formally known as Familial Cutaneous Aleeopathy (FCA) is an extremely rare genetic condition characterized by the development of skin lesions on the cheeks, extremities and upper torso. With no available cure, individuals affected by this disease develop unique challenges that can cause difficulty throughout their daily lives. Fortunately, there are resources available to those living with Pringles Disease that can help provide support, knowledge, and information.

The Pringles Disease Foundation: Established in 2015 by a group of Pringles Disease patients and their families, the Pringles Disease Foundation is dedicated to helping Pringles Disease families and educating the public on the condition. This organization advocates for early diagnosis and better understanding of the disease both socially and medically. Resources offered by the Pringles Disease Foundation include patient support, research and advocacy, care information, and access to a community of other Pringles Disease families.

Familial Cutaneous Aleeopathy International Database (FCAID): A resource created for medical professionals and designed to further the understanding of the genetic components of Pringles Disease. The FCAID links registered researchers from around the world to gather and share information, resources, and data. In addition, FCAID also serves to provide medical advice and guidance to healthcare professionals, as well as support to Pringles Disease patients and their families.

Global Genes: Global Genes is an organization that serves to spread awareness and understanding of Pringles Disease on a global basis. This organization sponsors events, educates advocacy groups, and facilitates partnerships among global leaders in Pringles Disease research. Global Genes also offers a variety of resources such as patient support groups, medical research tools, and rare disease-related news.

Pringles Disease Network: This online support group serves as a platform for sharing news, stories, and advice related to life with Pringles Disease. Pringles Disease Network is a safe and supportive environment for individuals with Pringles Disease to commune and connects, offering understanding, support, and friendship.

These are just a few of the resources available for individuals living with Pringles Disease and their families. For more information, please reach out to any of the organizations listed above or consult a doctor or genetic counselor for further questions and advice.

Conclusion

Our research has shown that Pringles Disease is a rare but serious condition that can have serious consequences if it is not properly diagnosed and treated. It can cause lifelong impairment and even death when left untreated. We have also seen how early diagnosis and proper medical care can help individuals with Pringles Disease live normal and fulfilling lives. With this knowledge in hand, we can raise awareness and ensure that everyone is aware of this serious but rare condition so that they can seek help when needed.